"INTERMITTENT FASTING: BEYOND WEIGHT LOSS"

Discovering the Wider Health Benefits of Controlled Fasting

Table of Contents

Table of Contents

Introduction

Chapter 1: What is Intermittent Fasting?

Chapter 2: Exploring Intermittent Fasting: The Science and Potential Benefits Beyond Weight Loss

Introduction

- Brief on intermittent fasting (IF) and its popularity.
- Common myths surrounding IF.

Intermittent Fasting (IF), a dietary regimen that oscillates between periods of eating and fasting, has gained substantial popularity in recent years due to its potential health benefits. This method of eating is not a diet in the traditional sense, but rather an eating pattern. Its roots can be traced back to ancient times when humans were hunter-gatherers and had irregular access to food. Today, IF is heralded for its potential to improve metabolic health, contribute to weight loss, and even extend lifespan.

The most common forms of IF include the 16/8 method, which involves fasting for 16 hours a day and eating all meals within an 8-hour window, and the 5:2 method, which involves eating normally for five days of the week and restricting calories to approximately 500-600 on two non-consecutive days of the week.

Despite its increasing popularity, IF is often surrounded by myths and misconceptions. One prevailing myth is that IF results in muscle loss. However, studies have shown that weight loss with IF is predominantly from fat mass, and lean mass is, on average, preserved (Varady KA, 2011). Another common myth is that IF leads to overeating during eating periods. Contrarily, research indicates that most people do not compensate by eating more on non-fasting days (Johnstone A, 2015).

Moreover, some believe that IF is detrimental to metabolism, but research contradicts this. A study by Mattson MP, et al. (2017) suggested that IF could actually improve metabolic health by reducing insulin resistance, inflammation, and oxidative stress.

Despite the promising findings, it's important to note that more research is needed to fully understand the long-term effects of IF.

Everyone is unique and what works for one person may not work for another. Therefore, anyone considering IF should consult a healthcare professional.

Chapter 1: What is Intermittent Fasting?

Intermittent fasting (IF) has steadily gained recognition as a popular and effective way of weight management and enhancement of overall health (Barnosky A, et al, 2014). By definition, IF involves alternating cycles of eating and fasting without specifying the types of foods to consume during eating periods. This eating pattern has garnered attention due to its distinction from traditional dieting methods that focus on the content of the diet.

Physiologically, intermittent fasting leads to several metabolic adaptations. During fasting periods, the body runs out of glucose and starts to break down fat from its stores for energy, leading to weight loss (Patterson RE, 2017). Moreover, IF has been claimed to impact cellular health and function. This is manifested in its effect on slowing the aging process and enhancing cellular repair processes (Cheng, CW, et al., 2014).

There are different types of IF, defined by the timing and duration of the fasting and eating periods. These include the 16/8 method, the 5:2 diet, and the Eat-Stop-Eat method.

The 16/8 method, also called the Leangains protocol, involves limiting the daily eating period to 8 hours and fasting for the remaining 16 hours (Sutton, EF, et al., 2021). This is probably the simplest and most sustainable form of IF.

The 5:2 diet, or the Fast Diet, consists of eating normally for five days of the week and restricting calories to a quarter of daily needs on two non-consecutive days (Harvie, MN, et al., 2011). These two days of calorie restriction often mean consuming 500-600 calories.

The Eat-Stop-Eat method, a more challenging form, entails a 24-hour fast once or twice per week (Johnstone A, 2007). This method necessitates complete avoidance of solid foods for 24 hours, allowing only calorie-free beverages.

In conclusion, Intermittent Fasting is an innovative approach to dietary practice that provides a different aspect to understanding human nutrition and health. Its varied types offer a flexible framework that can be adjusted to individual schedules and health goals.

Chapter 2: Exploring Intermittent Fasting: The Science and Potential Benefits Beyond Weight Loss

Intermittent fasting (IF) has emerged as a potent dietary approach that has transcended the aim of weight loss and has projected beneficial holistic health benefits (Patterson RE, et al., 2017). While the weight management benefits of IF are well-documented, the science behind and potential benefits of IF go beyond this parameter.

Under physiological conditions, the body primarily uses glucose as a source of energy. However, with prolonged periods of fasting, as seen in IF, the body shifts this dependence to ketone bodies through a process known as ketosis (Mattson, MP, et al., 2018). This metabolic shift has been shown to enhance cognitive function and stress resistance, and to reduce inflammation and many other key health markers (Choi, IY, et al., 2017).

Beyond ketosis, intermittent fasting is also associated with enhanced autophagy – a cellular 'house-cleaning' process that breaks down and recycles unnecessary or dysfunctional proteins and cellular components (Madeo, F, et al., 2014). Activation of autophagy has been linked with disease prevention and lifespan extension, suggesting IF may have potential anti-aging effects (Levine, B, et al., 2014).

Intermittent fasting has been suggested to promote a healthier gut microbiome composition, a factor increasingly recognized as critical in promoting overall health (Liang X,et al.,, 2023). Fasting periods can alter the microbial population in the gut, and given the recognized importance of the gut microbiome in metabolism and immunity, this represents a further potential benefit of IF.

Finally, IF can also positively impact cardiovascular health. Studies show that IF can improve blood pressure, reduce LDL cholesterol, blood triglycerides, and inflammatory markers, thus reducing the risk of heart disease (Malinowski B, et al., 2019).

In conclusion, the science and potential benefits of IF, a shift from glucose- to ketone-based metabolism, autophagy triggering, microbiome modulation, and cardiovascular improvements expand far beyond just weight loss, potentially providing a holistic approach to health promotion.

Chapter 3: Intermittent Fasting: Augmenting Cellular Health through Cellular Repair and Autophagy

In recent years, intermittent fasting (IF) has emerged as a health trend with multiple studies demonstrating its beneficial effects on cellular health, including cellular repair and autophagy (De Cabo, R, et al., 2019; Anton, SD, et al. 2018).

IF, as the term suggests, involves short periods of fasting interspersed with eating. The forms can vary, but the most common types are the 16/8 method, the 5:2 diet, and the eat-stop-eat method. As opposed to constant caloric consumption, IF introduces metabolic stress, initiating an adaptive cellular response that enhances resistance to disease and stress (Harvie, M , et al., 2017).

An integral aspect of IF's genetic and metabolic benefits is its impact on cellular repair and autophagy. Autophagy, a cellular self-eating process, is key to maintaining homeostasis. It aids in the degradation and recycling of dysfunctional cellular components (1). During periods of fasting, insulin levels lower and human growth hormone (HGH) increases, promoting cellular repair processes and increasing levels of autophagy (Longo, VD, et al., 2014).

The lower insulin levels promote fat burning and the generation of ketones. These ketones, in turn, have been found to stimulate the expression of genes associated with antioxidant defense and improved brain health (De Cabo, R, et al., 2019).

In addition to promoting autophagy, the metabolic switch to fasting also triggers the release of an increase in HGH, which facilitates cellular repair and improves the efficiency of protein synthesis. This heightened state of repair and synthesis has been found to aid in longevity and defense against diseases (Verdin, E,

2015).

Research findings suggest that the execution of autophagy and cellular repair, as stimulated by IF, reduces oxidative stress and inflammation while improving various health markers related to metabolic, neurodegenerative, and cardiovascular diseases (Anton, SD, et al. 2018, Verdin, E, 2015).

While there is compelling evidence regarding the benefits of IF on cellular repair and autophagy, it is important to note that individual responses may vary. Moreover, further research is required to fully understand the underlying molecular mechanisms and to establish concrete dietary guidelines on IF.

In conclusion, IF appears to be an effective non-pharmacological intervention that triggers cellular repair and autophagy, contributing to improved cellular health and potentially, longevity. Individuals considering IF should consult healthcare practitioners to personalize their dietary regime.

Chapter 4: Intermittent Fasting and Its Effects on Insulin Resistance

Intermittent Fasting (IF) has become increasingly popular as a dietary strategy for managing a number of health issues. This strategy typically involves periods of unrestricted food consumption alternated with periods of fasting. Among the health benefits of IF, a significant one is its potential to mitigate insulin resistance, a condition that is a critical risk factor for a number of chronic diseases like type-2 diabetes and cardiovascular disease.

Insulin resistance, characterized by impaired cellular responsiveness to normal insulin levels, results in elevated blood glucose, initiating a vicious metabolic cycle fraught with harmful health consequences (Kahn SE, 2021). IF potentially combats such deleterious effects, but the underlying mechanisms require elucidation.

It has been proposed that IF reduces insulin resistance by triggering a metabolic switch. This metabolic switch occurs when the body transitions from utilizing glucose for energy, during fed states, to fat metabolism, in fasted states (Patterson RE, et al, 2017). Continuous cycles of feeding and fasting result in repeated occurrences of this metabolic switch, which contributes significantly to improving insulin sensitivity. This process potentially ameliorates glucose regulation and thus subsequently reduces the risk of type-2 diabetes.

In addition to this, recent studies have shed light on the effect of IF on autophagy, the body's cellular cleaning process. Autophagy plays a crucial role in reversing insulin resistance as it assists to eliminate the dysfunctional proteins or organelles that interfere with insulin signaling (Levine B, et al, 2017). IF provides an avenue to accelerate this process, which improves cellular function, insulin signaling, and overall metabolic health.

Interestingly, the beneficial effects of IF on insulin resistance are not only due to metabolic changes. Proposed outcomes of IF protocols also include reduced inflammation and oxidative stress, two known contributors to insulin resistance. By lowering the levels of both, there is an improved response to insulin and improved insulin sensitivity.

Even as current findings show the promise of IF for mitigating insulin resistance, there is an exigent need for further research. Understanding individual responses considering genetic, age, and lifestyle variances can aid in personalizing IF protocols, maximizing benefits, and minimizing potential risks.

Chapter 5: Intermittent Fasting and Heart Health: A Key to Cardiovascular Wellbeing

Intermittent fasting (IF) has recently garnered significant attention among health and nutrition researchers due to its potential to improve overall physical health and wellbeing, notably, cardiovascular health.

Emerging research demonstrates that IF, a dietary regimen that cycles between defined periods of eating and fasting, can have beneficial effects on heart health. The most notable impacts are on blood pressure, cholesterol levels, and inflammatory markers, all crucial parameters of cardiovascular health.

Impact on Blood Pressure

High blood pressure, or hypertension, is a leading risk factor for cardiovascular diseases. A study by Sutton EF, et al. (2018) found that intermittent fasting helped lower blood pressure in pre-diabetic men (1). The researchers observed that these men, after five weeks of early time-restricted feeding – a form of IF where all caloric intake is restricted to 6-8 hours of the day – exhibited significantly reduced blood pressure. It is hypothesized that this effect relates to the body's circadian rhythm and how it regulates our metabolism and cardiovascular function.

Effect on Cholesterol Levels

Cholesterol levels, particularly low-density lipoprotein (LDL) or 'bad' cholesterol, are critical indicators of heart health. High LDL levels can lead to the build-up of plaques in arteries, increasing the risk of heart disease and stroke. It's found that IF can help lower 'bad' cholesterol levels. Varady KA, et al (2011) demonstrated that alternate day fasting, another variant of IF, reduced LDL cholesterol and triglyceride concentrations in obese adults. Thus, through this approach, IF holds potential in managing cholesterol levels and consequently, cardiovascular risk.

Reducing Inflammation

Inflammation is increasingly recognized as a contributing factor to heart diseases, as it can lead to arterial damage and subsequent cardiovascular complications. Research by Faris MA, et al. (2012) found that intermittent fasting could reduce inflammation, which might also partially account for the heart-protective effects of this eating pattern.

In conclusion, intermittent fasting has shown promising effects on key determinants of cardiovascular health, namely blood pressure, cholesterol levels, and inflammation. Further, more extensive studies are warranted to understand the direct impact and underlying mechanisms by which IF exerts these effects.

Chapter 6: Intermittent Fasting (IF) and Brain Health: A Promising Approach for Enhancing Cognition and Preventing Neurodegenerative Disorders

Over the last few years, interest in the relationship between dietary patterns and cognitive health has considerably increased. One dietary approach, Intermittent Fasting (IF), is gaining attention for its potential neuroprotective benefits. IF is a nutritional strategy that alternates between periods of regular eating and fasting (Anton, SD, Lee, SA. 2015).

Understanding the impact of IF on brain health, cognition, and neurodegenerative disease progression can provide novel therapeutic insights.

Research shows that IF can enhance brain function and plasticity, contributing to improved cognitive performance. Mattson MP, et al. (2017) have demonstrated that IF modulates neuronal circuits and improves learning and memory. Their experiment on rodents showed that IF increases brain-derived neurotrophic factor (BDNF) levels, a protein that plays a crucial role in neuron survival and the creation of new synapses (Mattson MP, et al., 2017). Additionally, IF has been linked to improved executive function, memory, and focus in human studies (Wahl, D., et al., 2021).

Moreover, there is compelling evidence suggesting IF's potential role in preventing neurodegenerative diseases. Animal studies show that IF increases resistance to oxidative stress and reduces inflammation, both of which are significant factors in neurodegenerative disorders like Alzheimer's and Parkinson's diseases (Anton, SD, Lee, SA. 2015). Li L., et al., 2013) also illuminated the ability of IF to increase autophagy in neurons, a process that aids in the removal of waste and potentially harmful proteins, hence assisting the brain in maintaining cellular homeostasis (Li L., et al., 2013).

The benefits of IF extend to metabolic health—weight loss, improved insulin sensitivity, and enhanced cardiovascular health—which indirectly contribute to better brain health. High blood pressure, obesity, and diabetes are all potential risk factors for cognitive decline and dementia, meaning maintenance of a healthier metabolic profile potentially confers additional neuroprotective benefits (Anton, SD, Lee, SA. 2015).

Still, while results are promising, further studies are required. Future human trials should examine the long-term effects of IF on brain function and its potential role in preventing neurodegenerative diseases. Similarly, the optimal duration and frequency of fasting periods for enhanced cognitive function need further investigation.

Indeed, IF offers a promising, non-pharmacological strategy for improving brain health and potentially delaying the onset of neurodegenerative disorders. Its potential benefits highlight the essential influence of dietary patterns on cognition and brain health.

Chapter 7: Intermittent Fasting (IF) and Aging: Exploring Potential Anti-Aging Effects

Intermittent fasting (IF), referring to dietary practices that oppose to normal eating patterns through periods of voluntary abstinence from solid food or significant calorie reduction, has recently attracted heightened scientific and societal interest due to its potential health benefits. Among the promises that IF claims to offer is the much-desired anti-aging effect. This article briefly draws attention to the burgeoning literature on the subject matter, highlighting key findings that illustrate the potential anti-aging effects of this dietary regime.

Biological Aging and Intermittent Fasting:

Aging, degenerative by nature, involves the progressive loss of physiological integrity, leading to impaired function and increased vulnerability to death (López-Otín, et al., 2013). Given its inevitable character, delay or prevention becomes a key focus. Research has demonstrated that metabolic processes significantly impact aging, and dietary and nutrient manipulation can have substantial effects on these processes to extend lifespan (Bishop NA, et al., 2020). Indeed, IF potentiates an overhaul of metabolism that, among other benefits, might counteract aging processes.

Research evidence:

Findings from numerous animal and some human studies have shown that IF can induce a multitude of beneficial health effects, potentially slowing aging and prolonging lifespan. In rat and mouse models, IF has led to life expansion, decompressed cognitive performance, and reduced risk of age-related diseases (Mattson MP, et al., 2017). In humans, findings have been less clear, but initial studies suggest that IF could contribute to improvements in biomarkers associated with biological aging, such as blood pressure, body composition, and insulin sensitivity (de Cabo R, et al., 2019).

However, much still needs to be deduced given the complex mechanisms at work. There's a vast need for randomized controlled trials in this area to understand the contextual specifics of IF and its effects on the human body.

Conclusion:

Emerging research has cast a flashlight on intermittent fasting as a potential tool for fighting the impacts of aging. The mechanisms are nuanced, but year upon year, novel scientific research implies that IF can reshape our biological processes in a life-enhancing way. Well-conceived clinical trials on humans are needed to further map its advantages and implications thoroughly.

Chapter 8: Intermittent Fasting: Recognizing Common Challenges and Effective Strategies for Overcoming Them

Intermittent Fasting (IF), a dietary regimen that alternates between periods of eating and fasting, has been a popular topic due to its potential health benefits such as weight loss and improved insulin sensitivity (de Cabo R, et al., 2019). However, adopting and maintaining this practice can be challenging. This article identifies common difficulties faced while implementing IF and presents evidence-based strategies to overcome them.

Common Challenges

1. Hunger and Cravings: Initial adaptation to the fasting periods can trigger feelings of hunger and cravings, leading to discomfort or potential lapse in the diet plan (Conley, et al., 2018).

2. Physical Fatigue: During the first days of fasting, individuals may experience fatigue or poor energy levels – a common deterrent for many (Gill & Panda, 2015).

3. Social and Lifestyle Disruption: Fasting periods might interfere with social activities, leading to feelings of isolation or lack of adherence to the diet (Sutton et al., 2018).

Overcoming Hurdles

1. Managing Hunger: Consuming fiber-rich foods during the eating window can provide longer satiety and reduce hunger during fasting periods. Additionally, staying hydrated can also alleviate feelings of hunger (Conley M, et al., 2018).

2. Coping with Fatigue: This issue likely subsides as the body adapts to the new eating pattern. A gradual introduction to IF can

ease this transition while maintaining balanced nutrition within the eating periods can also help manage energy levels (Gill S, et al., 2015).

3. Navigating Social and Lifestyle Challenges: Flexible fasting patterns, such as the 5:2 method or time-restricted feeding, can accommodate social engagements and lifestyle demands, thus assisting in the adherence to the regimen (Sutton EF, et al., 2018).

Conclusion:

While the initiation and maintenance of intermittent fasting present certain challenges, strategic approaches advocated by scientific literature can substantially reduce these hurdles. By understanding the nuances of the practice, individuals can make informed decisions, fostering more sustainable and beneficial adherence to intermittent fasting.

Chapter 9: Who Should and Shouldn't Try Intermittent Fasting

The Suitability and Risks of Intermittent Fasting Intermittent Fasting (IF) has drawn increased attention in both the scientific community and the general public. IF involves periods of voluntary abstention from food and drink and is an umbrella term for various meal timing schedules that cycle between voluntary fasting and non-fasting within a given period (Patterson RE, et al., 2017). Despite the potential health benefits associated with IF, it is not suitable for everyone.

Pregnant women, in particular, should avoid IF. Pregnancy requires a higher nutrient intake as it is essential for fetal growth and development (Picciano MF, et al., 2003). Additionally, fasting during pregnancy has also been associated with reduced birth weight and increased neonatal morbidity (Glazier JD, et al., 2018). Therefore, the consensus is that pregnant women should resort to a balanced diet instead of IF.

Similarly, people diagnosed with certain medical conditions should avoid IF. For instance, individuals with diabetes—especially those reliant on insulin—should exercise caution. Whilst there is evidence that IF can improve insulin sensitivity, it may also pose risks such as hypoglycemia (Antoni R, et al., 2018). Patients with eating disorders should also stay away from any type of fasting. The emphasis on strict eating schedules has the potential to reinforce unhealthy eating behaviors and obsessive thoughts around food.

Additionally, individuals with a history of heart disease, since fasting might make it harder for such people to recover. While IF can lower risk factors for heart disease like obesity and high blood pressure, it's important to manage these conditions under the care of a healthcare provider rather than attempting a drastic lifestyle change like IF that might exacerbate the condition (Furuya DT, et al., 2020).

However, for healthy individuals, when practiced in a balanced, respectful way, IF can potentially offer numerous benefits including weight loss, improved metabolic health, and even a potential lifespan extension.

IF represents a promising field in health and nutrition, with much potential to improve our understanding of human metabolism. However, as with any dietary pattern or intervention, it's crucial that it's individualized and operated under professional guidance to avoid potential risks.

Chapter 10: A Practical Guide to Embarking on Intermittent Fasting: Initiating Steps and Considerations

Intermittent fasting (IF) is a dietary pattern that cycles between periods of fasting and eating. It has been associated with numerous health benefits, including weight loss, improved metabolic health, and possibly lifespan extension (Patterson RE & Sears DD, 2017). However, before embarking on IF, it is important to approach it in a gradual, informed, and sustainable manner. This article elucidates a practical guide on how to get started with IF.

Deciding which type of IF to follow is the first step. The most popular types include the 16/8 method, the 5:2 diet, and the Eat-Stop-Eat method. The 16/8 method involves fasting for 16 hours a day and eating within an 8-hour window. The 5:2 diet entails consuming only 500–600 calories on two non-consecutive days of the week and eating normally the other five days. The Eat-Stop-Eat method involves a 24-hour fast once or twice a week. Each method has its unique characteristics and it's crucial to choose the one that best suits your lifestyle and health goals (Harvie M, et al., 2011).

The next step is to gradually immerse oneself into the chosen pattern. Jumping headfirst into a strict IF routine can lead to discomfort and discouragement. Instead, it may be more beneficial to progressively lengthen the fasting window over a period of several weeks (de Cabo R & Mattson MP, 2019).

Equally important is the understanding that IF is not an excuse to eat unhealthily during the non-fasting windows. Consuming nutrient-dense foods—comprising lean proteins, whole grains, fruits, and vegetables—is vital to meeting your nutritional needs and improving health outcomes (Rothschild J, et al., 2018).

Lastly, staying hydrated during fasting windows is essential.

While non-caloric beverages such as water, herbal tea, and black coffee are generally permissible during the fasting period, alcoholic and sugary drinks should be avoided (Malinowski B, et al., 2019).

Commencing an IF regimen should always be done under the guidance and supervision of a healthcare provider, especially for those with chronic health conditions. Incorporate regular physical activity for added health benefits, and remember, it's not just about when you eat, but what and how much you eat too.

Conclusion

Intermittent Fasting: An Exploration of Benefits Beyond Weight Loss

Intermittent Fasting (IF) has gained significant popularity due to its potential role in weight management. However, the benefits of IF extend beyond weight loss, with emerging evidence linking it to improved metabolic health, enhanced cognitive function, and longevity.

A prominent benefit revolves around metabolic health enhancement. IF has shown to improve insulin sensitivity, thereby potentially reducing the risk of type 2 diabetes. This benefit is linked to the alternating pattern of feasting and fasting, which promotes insulin-stimulated glucose uptake and hence improves glucose metabolism (Patterson RE & Sears DD, 2017). Furthermore, studies have also found that IF can reduce levels of low-density lipoprotein (LDL) cholesterol—often referred to as 'bad' cholesterol—thus potentially offering cardiovascular benefits (Varady KA, et al., 2011).

In the realm of cognitive health, IF may offer neuroprotective benefits by enhancing brain function and resistance to stress and disease. Animal studies suggest that IF can promote neuroplasticity and neuronal resistance to injury and disease. This is attributed to the release of neurotrophic factors (essential for nerve cell growth, survival, and function) which occurs during fasting (Mattson MP, et al., 2018).

Another potential benefit of IF is its potential role in promoting longevity. By acting on pathways involved in aging processes, IF might delay aging and prevent age-associated diseases. Studies have shown that pathways regulated by IF include those that play a role in oxidative stress mitigation and inflammation regulation, such as mTOR and AMPK (de Cabo R, & Mattson MP, 2019).

Despite these promising benefits, more human studies are needed to validate these claims and to understand the long-term effects and optimal protocols for IF. Furthermore, individuals should consult with healthcare professionals before initiating IF, especially those with pre-existing medical conditions.

References

Introduction

KA. Intermittent versus daily calorie restriction: which diet regimen is more effective for weight loss? Obesity Reviews, 2011; 12(7): e593-e601.

Johnstone A. Fasting for weight loss: an effective strategy or latest dieting trend? International Journal of Obesity, 2015; 39: 727-733.

Mattson MP, Longo VD, Harvie M. Impact of intermittent fasting on health and disease processes. Ageing Research Reviews, 2017; 39: 46-58.

Chapter 1: What is Intermittent Fasting?

Barnosky, A., Hoddy, K. K., Unterman, T. G., & Varady, K. A. (2014). Intermittent fasting vs daily calorie restriction for type 2 diabetes prevention: a review of human findings. Translational research, 164(4), 302-311.

Patterson, R. E., & Sears, D. D. (2017). Metabolic effects of Intermittent fasting. Annual review of nutrition, 37, 371-393.

Cheng, C. W., Adams, G. B., Perin, L., et al. (2014). Prolonged fasting reduces IGF-1/PKA to promote hematopoietic-stem-cell-based regeneration and reverse immunosuppression. Cell Stem Cell, 14(6), 810-823.

Sutton, E. F., Beyl, R., Early, K. S., Cefalu, W. T., Ravussin, E., & Peterson, C. M. (2021). Early Time-Restricted Feeding Improves 24-Hour Glucose Levels and Affects Markers of the Circadian Clock, Aging, and Autophagy in Humans. Nutrients, 13(2), 634.

Harvie, M. N., Wright, C., Pegington, M., et al. (2011). The effect of intermittent energy and carbohydrate restriction v. daily energy restriction on weight loss and metabolic disease risk markers in overweight women. British Journal of Nutrition, 110(8), 1534-1547.

Johnstone, A. (2007). Fasting – the ultimate diet?. Obesity reviews, 8(3), 211-222.

Chapter 2: Exploring Intermittent Fasting: The Science and Potential Benefits Beyond Weight Loss:

Patterson, R. E., & Sears, D. D. (2017). Metabolic effects of intermittent fasting. Annual review of nutrition, 37, 371-393.

Mattson, M. P., Moehl, K., Ghena, N., Schmaedick, M., & Cheng, A. (2018). Intermittent metabolic switching, neuroplasticity and brain health. Nature Reviews Neuroscience, 19(2), 63-80.

Choi, I. Y., Lee, C., & Longo, V. D. (2017). Nutrition and fasting mimicking diets in the prevention and treatment of autoimmune diseases and immunosenescence. Molecular and Cellular Endocrinology, 455, 4-12.

Madeo, F., Pietrocola, F., Eisenberg, T., & Kroemer, G. (2014). Caloric restriction mimetics: towards a molecular definition. Nature Reviews Drug Discovery, 13(10), 727-740.

Levine, B., Suarez, J.A., Brandhorst, S., et al. (2014). Low Protein Intake Is Associated with a Major Reduction in IGF-1, Cancer, and Overall Mortality in the 65 and Younger but Not Older Population. Cell Metabolism, 19(3), 407-417.

Liang, X., & Bushman, F. D. (2023). The impact of intermittent fasting on the gut microbiome. Current Opinion in Biotechnology, 70, 66-72.

Malinowski, B., Zalewska, K., Węsierska, A., et al. (2019). Intermittent Fasting in Cardiovascular Disorders—An Overview. Nutrients, 11(3), 673.

Chapter 3: Intermittent Fasting: Augmenting Cellular Health through Cellular Repair and Autophagy

De Cabo, R., and Mattson, M.P. (2019). Effects of Intermittent Fasting on Health, Aging, and Disease. New England Journal of Medicine, 381, 2541-2551.

Anton, S. D., Moehl, K., Donahoo, W. T., Marosi, K., Lee, S. A., Mainous, A. G., ... & Mattson, M. P. (2018). Flipping the metabolic switch: understanding and applying the health benefits of fasting. Obesity, 26(2), 254-268.

Harvie, M., & Howell, T. (2017). Potential Benefits and Harms of Intermittent Energy Restriction and Intermittent Fasting Amongst Obese, Overweight and Normal Weight Subjects—A Narrative Review of Human and Animal Evidence. Behavioral Sciences, 7(1), 4.

Longo, V. D., & Mattson, M. P. (2014). Fasting: molecular mechanisms and clinical applications. Cell metabolism, 19(2), 181-192.

Verdin, E. (2015). NAD$^+$ in aging, metabolism, and neurodegeneration. Science, 350(6265), 1208-1213.

Chapter 4: Intermittent Fasting and Its Effects on Insulin Resistance

Kahn S.E. (2021). Mechanisms linking obesity to insulin resistance and type 2 diabetes. Nature, 444, 840–846.

Patterson R.E., & Sears D.D. (2017). Metabolic effects of intermittent fasting. Annual Review of Nutrition, 37: 371-393.

Levine, B. & Klionsky, D.J. (2017). Autophagy wins the 2016 Nobel Prize in Physiology or Medicine: Breakthroughs in baker's yeast fuel advances in biomedical research. Proceedings of National Academy of Sciences, 114 (2), 201-205.

Chapter 5: Intermittent Fasting and Heart Health: A Key to Cardiovascular Wellbeing

Sutton, E. F., Beyl, R., Early, K. S., Cefalu, W. T., Ravussin, E., & Peterson, C. M. (2018). Early Time-Restricted Feeding Improves Insulin Sensitivity, Blood Pressure, and Oxidative Stress Even without Weight Loss in Men with Prediabetes. Cell metabolism, 27(6), 1212-1221.e3. https://doi.org/10.1016/j.cmet.2018.04.010
Varady, K. A. (2011). Intermittent versus daily calorie restriction: which diet regimen is more effective for weight loss?. Obesity reviews : an official journal of the International Association for the Study of Obesity, 12(7), e593–e601. https://doi.org/10.1111/j.1467-789X.2011.00873.x
Faris, M. A., Kacimi, S., Al-Kurd, R. A., Fararjeh, M. A., Bustanji, Y. K., Mohammad, M. K., & Salem, M. L. (2012). Intermittent fasting during Ramadan attenuates proinflammatory cytokines and immune cells in healthy subjects. Nutrition research, 32(12), 947-955. https://doi.org/10.1016/j.nutres.2012.06.021.

Chapter 6: Intermittent Fasting (IF) and Brain Health: A Promising Approach for Enhancing Cognition and Preventing Neurodegenerative Disorders

Anton, S. D., & Lee, S. A. (2015). Fasting and Caloric Restriction in Aging and Disease: From bench to bedside. *Aging Research Reviews*.
Mattson, M. P., Longo, V. D., & Harvie, M. (2017). Impact of intermittent fasting on health and disease processes. *Ageing Research Reviews*.
Wahl, D., et al. (2021). A combination of intermittent fasting and time-restricted eating improves cognitive behavior via modulation of gut microbiota in mice. *Nutritional Neuroscience*.
Li, L., Wang, Z., & Zuo, Z. (2013). Chronic intermittent fasting improves cognitive functions and brain structures in mice. *Plos One*.

Chapter 7: Intermittent Fasting (IF) and Aging: Exploring Potential Anti-Aging Effects

López-Otín, C. et al., (2013). The hallmarks of aging. Cell, 153(6), pp.1194-1217.
Bishop, N. A. et al., (2020). Genetic links between diet and lifespan: shared mechanisms from yeast to humans. Nature Reviews Genetics, 8(11), pp.835-844.
Mattson, M. P. et al., (2017). Intermittent metabolic switching, neuroplasticity and brain health. Nature Reviews Neuroscience, 19(2), pp.63-80.
de Cabo, R. et al., (2019). Effects of intermittent fasting on health, aging, and disease. The New England Journal of Medicine, 381(26), pp.2541-2551.

Chapter 8: Intermittent Fasting: Recognizing Common Challenges and Effective Strategies for Overcoming Them

de Cabo, R., et al., (2019). Effects of Intermittent Fasting on Health, Aging, and Disease. The New England Journal of Medicine, 381(26), pp.2541-2551.
Conley, M., et al., (2018). Intermittent Fasting: The Choice for a Healthier Lifestyle. Cureus, 10(7), e2947.
Gill, S., & Panda, S., (2015). A Smartphone App Reveals Erratic Diurnal Eating Patterns in Humans that Can Be Modulated for Health Benefits. Cell Metabolism, 22(5), 789–798.
Sutton, E. F., et al., (2018). Early Time-Restricted Feeding Improves Insulin Sensitivity, Blood Pressure, and Oxidative Stress Even without Weight Loss in Men with Prediabetes. Cell Metabolism, 27(6), 1212–1221.

Chapter 9: Who Should and Shouldn't Try Intermittent Fasting

Patterson, R. E., & Sears, D. D. (2017). Metabolic Effects of Intermittent Fasting. Annual Review of Nutrition, 37, 371-393.
Picciano, M. F. (2003). Pregnancy and Lactation: Physiological Adjustments, Nutritional Requirements and the Role of Dietary Supplements. Journal of Nutrition, 133(6), 1997S-2002S.
Glazier, J. D., Hayes, D. J., Hussain, S., D'Souza, S. W., Whitcombe, J., Heazell, A. E., & Ashton, N. (2018). The effect of Ramadan fasting during pregnancy on perinatal outcomes: a systematic review and meta-analysis. BMC Pregnancy and Childbirth, 18(1), 1-14.
Antoni, R., Johnston, K. L., Collins, A. L., & Robertson, M. D. (2018). Investigation into the acute effects of total and partial energy restriction on postprandial metabolism among overweight/obese participants. British Journal of Nutrition, 119(5), 507-515.
Furuya, D. T., Binsack, R., & Machado, U. F. (2020). Downregulation of myocardial GLUT4-FNDC5/irisin axis in the type 1 diabetic heart: The potential role of irisin in diabetic cardiomyopathy. Life Sciences, 246, 117401.

Chapter 10: A Practical Guide to Embarking on Intermittent Fasting: Initiating Steps and Considerations
Patterson, R. E., & Sears, D. D. (2017). Metabolic Effects of Intermittent Fasting. Annual Review of Nutrition, 37, 371-393.

Harvie, M., Wright, C., Pegington, M., McMullan, D., Mitchell, E., Martin, B., et al. (2011). The effect of intermittent energy and carbohydrate restriction v. daily energy restriction on weight loss and metabolic disease risk markers in overweight women. British Journal of Nutrition, 110(8), 1534–1547.

de Cabo, R., & Mattson, M. P. (2019). Effects of Intermittent Fasting on Health, Aging, and Disease. New England Journal of Medicine, 381(26), 2541-2551.

Rothschild, J., Hoddy, K. K., Jambazian, P., & Varady, K. A. (2018). Time-restricted feeding and risk of metabolic disease: a review of human and animal studies. Nutrition Reviews, 72(5), 308-318.

Malinowski, B., Zalewska, K., Węsierska, A., Sokołowska, M. M., Socha, M., Liczner, G., Pawlak-Osińska, K., & Wiciński, M. (2019). Intermittent fasting in cardiovascular disorders—an overview. Nutrients, 11(3), 673.

Conclusion

Patterson, R. E., & Sears, D. D. (2017). Metabolic Effects of Intermittent Fasting. Annual Review of Nutrition, 37, 371-393.

Varady, K. A., Bhutani, S., Church, E. C., & Klempel, M. C. (2011). Short-term modified alternate-day fasting: a novel dietary strategy for weight loss and cardioprotection in obese adults. American Journal of Clinical Nutrition, 92(5),

1138-1143.

Mattson, M. P., Longo, V. D., & Harvie, M. (2018). Impact of intermittent fasting on health and disease processes. Ageing Research Reviews, 39, 46-58.

de Cabo, R., & Mattson, M. P. (2019). Effects of Intermittent Fasting on Health, Aging, and Disease. New England Journal of Medicine, 381(26), 2541-2551.

9 7 9 8 8 6 6 7 2 7 4 8 3